Rhabdomyolysis

Pathogenesis, Diagnosis, and Treatment

Murphy Green

Table of Content

Chapter One

Introduction to Rhabdomyolysis

A complex medical condition known as rhabdomyolysis is characterized by the quick disintegration of injured or damaged skeletal muscle tissue, which releases intracellular muscle constituents into the bloodstream and extracellular space. These constituents include myoglobin, creatine kinase (CK), aldolase, lactate dehydrogenase, and electrolytes. There are several reasons why skeletal muscle integrity might be disrupted, such as infections, genetic abnormalities, direct muscle injury, and some drugs.

Because of the potential for consequences such as acute kidney injury, electrolyte imbalances, and disseminated intravascular coagulation, the disease may be fatal.

Rhabdomyolysis is thought to be caused by direct invasion and toxic degradation of muscle fibers, with possible involvement from infectious organisms such as bacteria, viruses, and parasites.

Among the frequent reasons for rhabdomyolysis are:

- Trauma
- Ischemia
- Medications
- Hazardous substances
- metabolic illnesses
- infections

There is a wide range of symptoms that can accompany rhabdomyolysis, such as reddish-brown urine, weakness, and muscle discomfort. Typically, blood tests for muscle proteins, such as creatine kinase, are used to confirm the diagnosis.

In order to avoid problems and enhance patient outcomes, early identification and treatment are crucial. Correction of fluid and electrolyte imbalances is the mainstay of rhabdomyolysis care, and supportive measures frequently result in positive clinical outcomes, particularly in youngsters.

1.1 Symptoms of rhabdomyolysis

The disorder known as rhabdomyolysis is characterized by the breakdown of muscle fibers, which allows the blood to include the protein known as myoglobin. Numerous symptoms and, sometimes, fatal complications may result from this illness. Among the typical signs of rhabdomyolysis are:

1. Pain and stiffness in the muscles: Patients frequently complain of pain and stiffness in the muscles, which may indicate underlying muscular damage.

2. Weakness: Patients may feel weakness in their trunk and limbs as a result of the breakdown of muscle fibers.

3. Swelling: Fluid buildup in the impacted muscles might result in swelling.

4. Dark urine: Myoglobinuria may be indicated by dark urine, which is a result of muscle fiber breakdown.

5. Kidney issues: Myoglobinuria may put the kidneys under pressure to remove waste from the blood, which may result in renal damage.

6. Digestive problems: Myoglobin leakage into the digestive tract can cause nausea, vomiting, and gastrointestinal pain in patients.

7. Cardiac arrhythmia: Abnormal cardiac rhythms can result from muscle fiber degradation.

8. Low blood pressure: A decrease in blood volume brought on by a loss of muscle function may result in a dip in blood pressure.

9. Fever: Fever can be brought on by inflammation and muscular tissue damage.

10. Disorientation and confusion: Myoglobin release into the bloodstream can result in disorientation and confusion, which may be a sign of renal failure or other issues.

If you encounter any of these signs, you must get medical help right away since rhabdomyolysis can be a potentially fatal illness that needs to be treated quickly.

1.2 Diagnostic procedures and blood tests

The diagnosis of rhabdomyolysis is mostly dependent on diagnostic techniques and blood testing. Healthcare professionals may use a number of tests to confirm the diagnosis and gauge the severity of rhabdomyolysis when it is suspected. Among the most important blood tests and diagnostic procedures are:

1. Creatine Kinase (CK) Levels: The muscles contain the enzyme CK. Increased blood levels of CK can be a marker of muscular injury, and rhabdomyolysis is frequently associated with noticeably high levels of CK.

2. Myoglobin Levels: A protein that is expelled from injured muscle cells is called myoglobin. A rise in myoglobin levels may result in myoglobinuria, which gives the urine a dark or

reddish-brown color. Rhabdomyolysis diagnosis can be aided by measuring myoglobin levels in the blood and urine.

3. Renal Function Tests: Myoglobin released during rhabdomyolysis can cause kidney injury. Thus, in order to evaluate kidney function and identify any possible renal damage, tests including blood urea nitrogen (BUN) and creatinine levels are carried out.

4. Electrolyte Levels: Calcium, phosphate, and potassium imbalances are among the electrolytes that can be brought on by rhabdomyolysis. These electrolyte imbalances are monitored and treated by blood tests, which can be crucial in the treatment of rhabdomyolysis.

5. Liver Function Testing: Since rhabdomyolysis can harm the liver, liver function testing may be carried out to gauge the condition's overall effect on the body.

6. Urinalysis: Tests on urine are carried out to determine whether myoglobin is present and

how it affects the kidneys. One major sign of rhabdomyolysis is the distinctive reddish-brown color of the urine caused by myoglobinuria.

Confirming the diagnosis of rhabdomyolysis, determining its severity, and keeping an eye on its related complications—particularly kidney damage—all depend on these diagnostic techniques and blood tests. In order to manage rhabdomyolysis and avoid potential consequences, prompt and suitable treatment must be started after an early and precise diagnosis.

1.3 Differential diagnosis

When making a differential diagnosis for rhabdomyolysis, one must take into account other illnesses that may manifest with the same symptoms and test results. Because rhabdomyolysis can present with a wide range of symptoms and risk factors, the diagnosis is made using a combination of clinical examination and laboratory investigations. Several crucial elements of the diagnostic techniques and differential diagnosis for rhabdomyolysis encompass:

1. Clinical Assessment: To determine probable causes and risk factors for rhabdomyolysis, a complete history and physical examination are necessary. Individuals who have experienced trauma, infections, immobilization, or muscular illness are more susceptible to rhabdomyolysis and should be suspected of having it.

2. Laboratory Tests: One of the main indicators of rhabdomyolysis is elevated serum creatine kinase (CK) levels. Furthermore, rhabdomyolysis causes noticeably higher urine myoglobin levels, which might result in myoglobinuria and black urine. Confirming the diagnosis requires these tests.

3. Renal Function Tests: Blood urea nitrogen (BUN) and creatinine levels are tested to evaluate kidney function and identify any possible kidney damage because rhabdomyolysis can cause acute kidney injury due to the release of myoglobin.

4. Electrolyte Levels: Calcium, phosphate, and potassium imbalances are among the electrolytes that can be brought on by rhabdomyolysis. These electrolyte imbalances are monitored and treated by blood tests, which can be crucial in the treatment of rhabdomyolysis.

5. Urinalysis: Tests on urine are carried out to determine whether myoglobin is present and how it affects the kidneys. One major sign of rhabdomyolysis is the distinctive reddish-brown color of the urine caused by myoglobinuria.

6. Muscle Biopsy and Genetic Testing: In certain circumstances, particularly in individuals with recurrent rhabdomyolysis or when an acquired cause is difficult to determine, muscle biopsy and genetic testing may be taken into consideration.

7. Other illnesses: In addition to rhabdomyolysis, illnesses like myocardial infarction, influenza, and fibromyalgia may also

be taken into account during the differential diagnosis process.

To sum up, a thorough approach involving clinical evaluation, laboratory testing, and examination of other illnesses that may present similarly is required for the differential diagnosis of rhabdomyolysis. Accurately identifying rhabdomyolysis and distinguishing it from other possible causes of muscle damage and associated symptoms requires the use of this method.

Chapter Two

Pathogenesis

A complex medical disorder known as rhabdomyolysis is defined by the quick disintegration of injured or damaged skeletal muscle, which releases intracellular components of the muscle into the extracellular space and bloodstream. These components include myoglobin, creatine kinase (CK), aldolase, and electrolytes. Numerous causes of muscle injury, such as trauma, muscular ischemia, infections, toxins, medications, disorders of the electrolyte and metabolic system, genetic disorders, effort, extended bed rest, and temperature-induced states, can start this process. Acute renal failure, disseminated intravascular coagulation, and electrolyte imbalances are just a few of the consequences that can arise from the breakdown of skeletal muscle integrity and the consequent release of myoglobin.

The following crucial elements are involved in the pathophysiology of rhabdomyolysis:

1. Muscle Damage: Rhabdomyolysis, which releases intracellular muscle components into the bloodstream, can be triggered by any type of muscle damage, traumatic or non-traumatic.

2. Myoglobin Release: Myoglobinuria, a condition where myoglobin is present in the urine and gives it a distinctive red or brown hue, is caused by the release of myoglobin from injured muscle cells, which is a hallmark of rhabdomyolysis.

3. Renal Complications: Myoglobin can block the renal tubules and induce renal damage, which can result in acute kidney injury when it is present in the bloodstream.

4. Systemic repercussions: Rhabdomyolysis may have systemic repercussions, such as the possibility of electrolyte imbalances and disseminated intravascular coagulation, which may exacerbate the condition's complications.

The clinical examination, history, and laboratory tests, such as blood creatine kinase and urine myoglobin levels, are essential in the diagnostic evaluation of rhabdomyolysis because they confirm the diagnosis and determine the severity of the illness. Genetic testing and muscle biopsy may be used to find underlying genetic causes or intrinsic variables causing the illness in cases of recurrent rhabdomyolysis.

In conclusion, the pathophysiology of rhabdomyolysis includes the possibility of renal and systemic problems, the quick disintegration of injured muscle, and the release of myoglobin and other intracellular muscle components. The correct diagnosis and treatment of rhabdomyolysis depend on an understanding of its underlying mechanisms and causes.

2.1 Muscle injury and breakdown

Intracellular muscle components are released as a result of muscle injury and breakdown in rhabdomyolysis, which can cause a number of systemic problems. Rapid dissolution of damaged or injured skeletal muscle is a pathophysiology of rhabdomyolysis. This dissolution can be caused by a variety of reasons, including trauma, muscle compression, metabolic and electrolyte abnormalities, medications, toxins, and genetic defects. Intracellular muscle components, such as myoglobin, creatine kinase (CK), aldolase, and electrolytes, are directly released into the circulation and extracellular space when the integrity of the skeletal muscle is compromised.

Myoglobin, CK, and other intracellular materials can leak into the extracellular fluid as a result of acute trauma or metabolic imbalances that cause muscle damage and breakdown in rhabdomyolysis. Acute kidney damage and systemic inflammatory response are among the consequences that may result from this process, which can also induce volume depletion, electrolyte imbalances, and potentially hazardous intracellular contents to leak into the systemic circulation.

Rhabdomyolysis has non-specific clinical features, meaning that symptoms like muscle soreness, weakness, and myoglobinuria-related dark urine might occur. Monitoring renal function and electrolyte imbalances, along with measuring muscle enzyme levels like CK and myoglobin, are all part of the diagnostic process for rhabdomyolysis.

To summarize, the pathophysiology of rhabdomyolysis entails the quick breakdown of injured skeletal muscle, which releases intracellular muscle components and raises the risk of systemic side effects, especially acute kidney injury. Accurate diagnosis and treatment of rhabdomyolysis depend on an understanding of the fundamental principles of muscle damage and breakdown.

2.2 Genetic and acquired causes

Both hereditary and acquired causes can result in rhabdomyolysis, which causes injured or damaged skeletal muscle to dissolve quickly. A mix of environmental stressors and genetic predispositions often contribute to the multifactorial nature of the disorder. The following are some of the main hereditary and acquired causes of rhabdomyolysis:

1. hereditary susceptibility: Due to hereditary variables affecting muscle integrity and function, certain people may be predisposed to rhabdomyolysis from birth. Rhabdomyolysis can arise as a result of genetic illnesses such as mitochondrial myopathies, metabolic myopathies, and muscular dystrophies.

2. External Triggers: Physical activity, trauma, drug or alcohol misuse, infections, muscular ischemia, electrolyte and metabolic problems, usage of specific drugs, and toxins are some examples of external triggers that can cause rhabdomyolysis events. These outside influences have the potential to cause muscle deterioration and injury, which could ultimately lead to the systemic release of intracellular muscle components.

3. Mitochondrial Disorders: Rhabdomyolysis may occasionally be linked to mitochondrial disorders, which can show up as a variety of extra-muscular symptoms, such as encephalopathies, cardiomyopathies, and endocrinopathies.

The diagnosis of rhabdomyolysis is determined by a thorough review that includes laboratory testing, history, and clinical examination. To find underlying genetic causes or intrinsic variables contributing to the illness, muscle biopsy and genetic testing may be used in cases of recurrent rhabdomyolysis.

In conclusion, there are both acquired and hereditary causes of rhabdomyolysis, and the disorder frequently results from a complicated interaction between hereditary vulnerability and environmental triggers. Accurate diagnosis and treatment of rhabdomyolysis depend on knowledge of the underlying acquired and hereditary variables.

2.3 Infectious, traumatic, and nontraumatic etiologies

Numerous viral, traumatic, and non-traumatic etiologies can result in Rhabdomyolysis. Physical compression, auto accidents, and crush traumas are examples of traumatizing causes of rhabdomyolysis that can result in muscle injury and breakdown. Rhabdomyolysis can result from non-traumatic causes such as imbalances in the supply and demand of oxygen, changes in electrolytes, and anomalies in metabolism. Rhabdomyolysis can also be brought on by medications like statins, corticosteroids, and antimalarials.

Rhabdomyolysis can be caused by bacterial and viral infections, including Streptococcus and Legionella, as well as coxsackievirus, HIV, and influenza. Intracellular muscle components may be released into the bloodstream as a result of these viruses' ability to cause muscle injury and breakdown.

Rhabdomyolysis can also arise as a result of metabolic and electrolyte imbalances, including hypokalemia, hyperkalemia, hypophosphatemia, and hypocalcemia [2]. These abnormalities may cause a breakdown and injury to the muscles, which may then cause the intracellular components of the muscles to leak into the blood.

Rhabdomyolysis can also arise as a result of genetic illnesses such as mitochondrial myopathies, metabolic myopathies, and muscular dystrophies. Muscular injury and breakdown may result from certain illnesses that impair muscular integrity and function.

In conclusion, a wide range of infectious, traumatic, and non-traumatic etiologies can result in rhabdomyolysis. The correct diagnosis and treatment of rhabdomyolysis depend on an understanding of its underlying causes. It takes a thorough diagnostic assessment, which includes a clinical examination, history, and laboratory testing, to determine the underlying cause of rhabdomyolysis and start the right course of treatment.

Chapter Three

Treatment and Management

The main goals of rhabdomyolysis treatment and management are to treat the underlying cause, avoid complications, and maintain renal function. Key components of rhabdomyolysis treatment and management include the following:

1. Fluid Resuscitation: To preserve urine output and avoid acute kidney injury, adequate fluid resuscitation is necessary. Intravenous fluids, usually isotonic saline, are injected into the kidneys to facilitate the removal of myoglobin and other harmful byproducts and to guarantee proper renal perfusion.

In order to effectively manage rhabdomyolysis, it is imperative to closely monitor and correct electrolyte imbalances, such as hyperkalemia and hypocalcemia. Elevations of electrolytes that are abnormal can worsen myopathy and cause heart problems.

3. Addressing Underlying Causes: It's critical to determine and treat the underlying cause of rhabdomyolysis. This could entail managing any traumatic or exertional factors that contributed to the disease, treating infections, resolving metabolic imbalances, and stopping or modifying medication.

4. Renal Function Monitoring: In order to evaluate renal function and identify any indications of acute kidney injury, renal function monitoring, including serum creatinine and urine output, must be done continuously. Renal replacement treatment might be necessary in extreme circumstances to maintain renal function.

5. Avoidance of Nephrotoxins: To prevent further kidney injury in patients with rhabdomyolysis, nephrotoxic substances such as non-steroidal anti-inflammatory medications (NSAIDs) and some antibiotics should be avoided.

6. Muscle Rest and Supportive Care: In order to speed up healing and stop more muscle

damage, patients with rhabdomyolysis may need to get supportive care and muscle rest. Bed rest and pain control may be necessary in this situation.

7. Consequences Monitoring: Prompt intervention and care are contingent upon vigilant observation for possible rhabdomyolysis consequences, including disseminated intravascular coagulation, compartment syndrome, and cardiac arrhythmias.

Rhabdomyolysis can be treated and managed by addressing the underlying cause, promoting renal function, resolving fluid and electrolyte imbalances, and keeping an eye out for any complications. Optimizing patient outcomes and preventing long-term problems requires a comprehensive approach that includes supportive care, electrolyte monitoring, and fluid resuscitation.

3.1 Early intervention and its importance

The management of rhabdomyolysis necessitates early intervention since fast diagnosis and treatment can enhance results and avoid complications. Important elements of rhabdomyolysis early intervention include the following:

1. Early Recognition: Timely diagnosis and treatment of rhabdomyolysis depend on early recognition of the condition. Individuals who have experienced trauma, infections, immobilization, or muscular illness are more susceptible to rhabdomyolysis and should be suspected of having it.

2. Diagnostic Evaluation: To determine the underlying cause of rhabdomyolysis and start the proper course of treatment, a thorough diagnostic evaluation that includes a clinical examination, history, and laboratory studies is required. Rhabdomyolysis is characterized by elevated blood creatine kinase (CK) and urine myoglobin levels.

3. Fluid Resuscitation: To sustain urine output and avoid severe kidney injury, adequate fluid resuscitation is necessary. Intravenous fluids, usually isotonic saline, are injected into the kidneys to facilitate the removal of myoglobin and other harmful byproducts and to guarantee proper renal perfusion.

The correction and close monitoring of electrolyte imbalances, including hypocalcemia and hyperkalemia, are essential in the management of rhabdomyolysis. Elevations of electrolytes that are abnormal can worsen myopathy and cause heart problems.

5. Addressing Underlying Causes: It's critical to determine and treat the underlying cause of rhabdomyolysis. This could entail managing any traumatic or exertional factors that contributed to the disease, treating infections, resolving metabolic imbalances, and stopping or modifying medication.

6. Renal Function Monitoring: To evaluate renal function and identify any indications of acute kidney injury, renal function monitoring,

including serum creatinine and urine output, is required on a continuous basis. Renal replacement treatment might be necessary in extreme circumstances to maintain renal function.

In conclusion, timely diagnosis and treatment are essential for the effective management of rhabdomyolysis since they can avert complications and enhance results. Early intervention in rhabdomyolysis involves a thorough diagnostic diagnosis, fluid resuscitation, electrolyte monitoring, and addressing underlying causes.

3.2 Fluid and electrolyte correction

Maintaining proper fluid and electrolyte balance is essential for managing rhabdomyolysis. Myoglobin, creatine kinase, and electrolytes—intracellular muscle components—are released into the bloodstream during rhabdomyolysis, a fast breakdown of muscle fibers. Acute kidney damage and disseminated intravascular coagulation are among the consequences that may result from this process, which can also induce volume depletion, electrolyte imbalances, and potentially hazardous intracellular contents to leak into the systemic circulation.

Maintaining proper hydration and electrolyte balance is the major objective of fluid and electrolyte correction in rhabdomyolysis in order to avoid severe kidney damage and associated consequences. Intravenous fluids, usually isotonic saline, are injected to guarantee sufficient renal perfusion and facilitate the kidneys' removal of myoglobin and other harmful waste products. To avoid cardiac problems and additional muscle injury, electrolyte imbalances such as hypocalcemia and hyperkalemia are continuously monitored and treated as necessary.

For effective care, addressing the underlying cause of rhabdomyolysis is crucial, in addition to correcting fluid and electrolyte imbalances. This could entail managing any traumatic or exertional factors that contributed to the disease, treating infections, resolving metabolic imbalances, and stopping or modifying medication.

To sum up, maintaining proper fluid and electrolyte balance is essential for managing rhabdomyolysis. To avoid acute kidney injury and associated consequences, it's crucial to maintain proper electrolyte balance and adequate hydration. Key elements of managing rhabdomyolysis include intravenous fluids, electrolyte monitoring, and correction.

3.3 Hospital admission and intravenous fluid therapy

Intravenous fluid treatment and hospital admission are essential components of rhabdomyolysis care. Patients are evaluated for respiration, circulation, and airway at the time of admission, and supportive care is given if required. The management of rhabdomyolysis requires the following elements of intravenous fluid therapy and hospital admission:

1. Intravenous Access: Using a large-bore catheter to obtain intravenous (IV) access is essential for giving fluids and medications.

2. Fluid Resuscitation: The first line of treatment for rhabdomyolysis is fluid resuscitation, which needs to start very soon. Normal saline or other isotonic fluids are given at a rate of about 400 mL/h. Hydration at a rate of two to three times per day may then be adequate.

3. Monitoring Urine Output: To carefully monitor urine output and identify any indications of acute kidney injury, a Foley catheter is inserted.

4. Addressing Underlying Causes: It's critical to determine and treat the underlying cause of rhabdomyolysis. This could entail managing any traumatic or exertional factors that contributed to the disease, treating infections, resolving metabolic imbalances, and stopping or modifying medication.

5. Electrolyte Monitoring: To avoid problems and preserve appropriate physiological function, careful monitoring of electrolyte levels, such as those of potassium, phosphate, and calcium, is necessary.

In conclusion, two essential components of treating rhabdomyolysis are hospital admission and intravenous fluid therapy. The therapy and management of rhabdomyolysis must include prompt identification, fluid resuscitation, urine output monitoring, addressing underlying causes, and electrolyte monitoring.

3.4 Monitoring for complications

It is essential to monitor for complications in rhabdomyolysis in order to avoid and treat any potential side effects of the disorder. The following are some of the main issues and monitoring techniques:

1. Compartment Syndrome: A dangerous side effect of rhabdomyolysis, compartment syndrome is defined by elevated pressure inside a confined fascial region, which causes

discomfort, edema, and impaired blood flow. Prompt intervention, such as fasciotomy, and close monitoring of compartment pressures are necessary to avoid long-term complications.

2. Acute Kidney Injury: Myoglobin and other intracellular muscle components released into the bloodstream during rhabdomyolysis can result in acute kidney injury. This can block the renal tubules and cause renal damage. It is essential to monitor renal function, including urine output and blood creatinine levels, in order to identify acute kidney injury early and start the proper treatment.

3. Disseminated Intravascular Coagulation: The creation of clots in small blood vessels is a life-threatening complication of disseminated intravascular coagulation (DIC), which can be facilitated by Rhabdomyolysis. Prompt diagnosis and treatment of diabetic foot infection (DIC) require vigilant monitoring for symptoms such as limb edema, bruising, and unexplained bleeding.

4. Cardiac Arrhythmias: The release of potassium from injured muscle cells resulting in hyperkalemia is a cause of cardiac arrhythmias caused by rhabdomyolysis. It is essential to keep an eye on potassium levels, in particular, to avoid heart problems and preserve healthy physiological function.

5. Infections: Due to the release of intracellular muscle components and the possibility of weakened immune systems, patients with rhabdomyolysis may be more susceptible to infections. For an early diagnosis and course of therapy, it is imperative to keep an eye out for symptoms of infection, such as fever, chills, and leukocytosis.

In conclusion, it is essential to keep an eye out for any complications related to rhabdomyolysis in order to avoid and treat the condition. For the purpose of early detection and treatment, close monitoring of renal function, electrolyte levels, and clinical infection symptoms is necessary.

Chapter Four

Complications and Prognosis

In cases of rhabdomyolysis, prognosis and complications are tightly associated because certain problems may have long-term effects and affect the patient's course of treatment. Among the main side effects and predictors of rhabdomyolysis are:

1. Acute Kidney Injury: Myoglobin and other intracellular muscle components released into the bloodstream during rhabdomyolysis can result in acute kidney injury. This can block the renal tubules and cause renal damage. Patients with rhabdomyolysis who develop acute kidney injury are at a higher risk of developing renal failure, which can have a substantial impact on the patient's long-term prognosis and necessitate dialysis.

2. Disseminated Intravascular Coagulation: The creation of clots in small blood vessels is a life-threatening complication of disseminated intravascular coagulation (DIC), which can be facilitated by rhabdomyolysis. Patients with

rhabdomyolysis have a worse prognosis when DIC develops because uncontrolled clotting can cause multi organ failure and have a major negative influence on the patient's long-term health.

3. Cardiac Arrhythmias: The release of potassium from injured muscle cells resulting in hyperkalemia is a cause of cardiac arrhythmias caused by rhabdomyolysis. Cardiac problems may significantly affect the prognosis and long-term results of the patient.

4. Infections: Due to the release of intracellular muscle components and the possibility of weakened immune systems, patients with rhabdomyolysis may be more susceptible to infections. The course of the patient's treatment and long-term results may be adversely affected by the emergence of infections.

5. Multisystem Organ Failure: Renal, cardiac, and respiratory failure are among the multisystem organ failures that can result from rhabdomyolysis. These failures can significantly

affect the patient's prognosis and long-term outcome.

In conclusion, prognosis and complications in rhabdomyolysis are tightly associated since certain problems may have long-term effects on the patient. Early intervention and better patient outcomes depend on closely monitoring for complications and treating underlying causes.

4.1 Acute kidney injury

Rapid skeletal muscle disintegration following injury or damage results in the release of intracellular muscle components into the bloodstream, which is the hallmark of the complicated medical illness known as rhabdomyolysis. An acute kidney injury (AKI) is one of the most dangerous side effects of rhabdomyolysis, and it affects a large proportion of patients. The three main pathophysiological mechanisms underlying renal damage in rhabdomyolysis are intratubular cast formation resulting from myoglobin precipitation, direct tubular toxicity, and renal vasoconstriction. In the context of rhabdomyolysis, the onset of AKI can significantly affect patient outcomes and death.

One of the main objectives of rhabdomyolysis treatment is to avoid acute renal damage. This entails intensive and prompt fluid resuscitation in order to preserve urine production and shield the kidneys. Myoglobin and other toxic byproducts are cleared from the kidneys, and adequate renal perfusion is ensured by administering intravenous fluid treatment with isotonic fluids, such as normal saline. It is crucial to closely monitor blood creatinine levels, urine output, and electrolyte balance in order to identify early indicators of acute renal injury and start the right treatment.

Patients with rhabdomyolysis who suffer acute kidney injury are at a higher risk of developing renal failure, which can have a substantial influence on the patient's long-term prognosis and necessitate dialysis. Therefore, the treatment of individuals with rhabdomyolysis must focus on early detection, diagnosis, and proactive management to prevent acute renal impairment.

In conclusion, preventing acute kidney injury is a major therapy objective because it is a significant consequence of rhabdomyolysis. Prompt management, regular monitoring of renal function, and aggressive early fluid resuscitation are crucial for managing acute kidney injury in rhabdomyolysis patients.

4.2 Electrolyte imbalances

Rhabdomyolysis is a medical disorder that causes damaged or injured skeletal muscle to dissolve quickly, releasing intracellular muscle components into the bloodstream. One typical consequence of this condition is electrolyte imbalances. Electrolyte abnormalities brought on by the release of these components may result in problems such as acute renal damage, seizures, and cardiac arrhythmias.

Electrolyte abnormalities such as hyperkalemia, hypocalcemia, and hyperphosphatemia are most frequently linked to rhabdomyolysis. A potentially fatal consequence that can cause cardiac arrhythmias and cardiac arrest is hyperkalemia. While hyperphosphatemia can result in severe renal damage and other consequences, hypocalcemia can produce seizures, tetany, and cramping in the muscles.

Monitoring electrolyte levels closely and correcting imbalances as soon as they occur are key components of managing electrolyte imbalances in rhabdomyolysis. Intravenous fluids, usually isotonic saline, are injected to guarantee sufficient renal perfusion and facilitate the kidneys' removal of myoglobin and other harmful waste products. To avoid cardiac problems and additional muscle injury, electrolyte imbalances such as hypocalcemia and hyperkalemia are continuously monitored and treated as necessary.

In conclusion, electrolyte imbalances are a frequent side effect of rhabdomyolysis that must be managed to avoid more problems and enhance patient outcomes. The management of rhabdomyolysis necessitates close monitoring of electrolyte levels and timely repair of any abnormalities.

4.3 Long-term muscle weakness and recovery

Significant characteristics of rhabdomyolysis include long-term muscle weakening and recuperation, which can affect the patient's functional abilities and quality of life. A medical disorder known as rhabdomyolysis is defined by the quick disintegration of skeletal muscle that has been wounded or damaged, releasing intracellular muscle components into the bloodstream. In addition to other symptoms, including cramps, stiffness, and swelling, this procedure may result in muscle soreness, weakening, and other side effects.

The disruption of the sarcolemma and the release of intracellular muscle contents, such as myoglobin, creatine kinase, aldolase, and lactate dehydrogenase, as well as electrolytes into the bloodstream and extracellular space, are linked to the pathophysiology of long-term muscle weakness in rhabdomyolysis. When muscle integrity is compromised, intracellular muscle components may be directly released, resulting in muscular injury and the potential for long-term muscle weakening and recovery.

A thorough medical history, physical examination, and the proper diagnostic tests—such as muscle biopsy and genetic testing—are necessary for the diagnosis of long-term muscle weakness and recovery in rhabdomyolysis. These diagnostic instruments can direct the creation of a suitable treatment plan and assist in determining the underlying cause of muscular weakness.

In order to treat and manage long-term muscle weakness and recovery in rhabdomyolysis, supportive care must be given, rehabilitation and physical therapy must be implemented, and the underlying cause must be addressed. Genetic testing may be helpful in determining the underlying causes of recurrent episodes of rhabdomyolysis, as these may reveal problems in muscle structure or metabolism.

In conclusion, significant features of rhabdomyolysis that may affect a patient's quality of life and functional capacities are long-term muscle weakening and recuperation. The underlying cause of long-term muscle weakening and recovery in rhabdomyolysis must be addressed in addition to offering supportive care and putting rehabilitation and physical therapy programs into place.

Chapter Five

Prevention and Outlook

Rapid skeletal muscle disintegration following injury or damage results in the release of intracellular muscle components into the bloodstream, which is the hallmark of the complicated medical illness known as rhabdomyolysis. Muscle cramps, stiffness, edema, and other symptoms may be brought on by this process in addition to muscle pain and weakening. Preventing rhabdomyolysis entails staying away from recognized triggers, including intense physical activity, specific pharmaceuticals, and illegal substances. Rhabdomyolysis can also be avoided by staying properly hydrated and avoiding dehydration when engaging in physically demanding activities.

If patients with rhabdomyolysis receive quick and proper treatment, their prognosis is usually favorable. However, the severity of the ailment, the existence of underlying medical disorders, and the emergence of complications like acute renal injury can all affect the prognosis. Patients with rhabdomyolysis require aggressive management, early detection, and diagnosis to avoid acute kidney damage.

To summarize, the management of rhabdomyolysis involves steering clear of recognized triggers and ensuring sufficient hydration, particularly during physically demanding activities. When rhabdomyolysis is treated promptly and appropriately, the prognosis is usually good; however, the severity of the ailment and the emergence of comorbidities can affect the prognosis.

5.1 Risk factors and preventive measures

Rhabdomyolysis Risk Factors and Preventive Steps

- **Danger Elements**

Although anyone can get rhabdomyolysis, there are some conditions that make it more likely to happen. Among them are:

Trauma: Rhabdomyolysis is frequently caused by direct muscular injury, such as that which occurs following a car accident or crush injury.

Overexertion: Rhabdomyolysis and muscular breakdown can result from excessive physical exercise, particularly in those who are not trained.

Medications: Rhabdomyolysis can be brought on by some medications, including antipsychotics, statins, and illegal substances like cocaine and amphetamines.

Infections: Rhabdomyolysis can result from bacterial and viral infections, particularly in severe cases.

Metabolic problems: People who have certain metabolic abnormalities, like mitochondrial myopathies and glycogen storage illnesses, are more likely to experience rhabdomyolysis.

- **Preventative Actions**

Recognizing and addressing the underlying risk factors is necessary to prevent rhabdomyolysis. Among the preventive actions are:

i. Steer clear of excessive physical exercise, especially for people who are not trained.
ii. Drinking enough water when exercising and in hot weather.

iii. keeping an eye on and controlling drugs that can result in rhabdomyolysis, particularly in people who are at high risk

iv. Taking care of metabolic issues and underlying infections.

v. Steer clear of alcohol and illegal drugs.

Timely identification and management of rhabdomyolysis is crucial in order to avert complications and enhance patient results. Do not delay in seeking medical assistance if you suspect rhabdomyolysis.

5.2 Prognosis and long-term outcomes

When rhabdomyolysis is treated promptly and appropriately, the prognosis is usually good, especially in children. Rhabdomyolysis patients have an overall death rate of about 5%. However, the underlying reason and any coexisting comorbidities affect a patient's chance of dying individually. Treatment approaches have decreased the condition's related morbidity and mortality.

Particularly in children, recurrent bouts of rhabdomyolysis may be a sign of underlying problems with muscle form or metabolism. As a result, the underlying etiology and the efficacy of interventions aimed at addressing the underlying cause may have an impact on the prognosis and long-term results in such cases.

Only 6% of patients in a 10-year retrospective pediatric analysis passed away, suggesting that pediatric patients generally had favorable prognosis. This emphasizes how crucial early detection, diagnosis, and treatment are to enhancing patient outcomes and averting long-term rhabdomyolysis-related complications.

Adults with rhabdomyolysis may have different long-term outcomes and prognoses based on the underlying etiology, the existence of comorbidities, and the prompt use of suitable treatment approaches. Therefore, maximizing long-term results and prognosis in affected patients requires a comprehensive approach to rhabdomyolysis care, including the identification and treatment of underlying causes.

Conclusion

In conclusion, rhabdomyolysis is a complicated medical condition that can be brought on by a number of things, such as injuries, infections, drugs, overexertion, and metabolic problems. Rhabdomyolysis can present with a variety of clinical symptoms, but common ones include weakness, discomfort in the muscles, and reddish-brown urine.

It is imperative to have an early diagnosis and treatment in order to avoid consequences like acute renal damage. Preventing acute kidney injury and maintaining appropriate fluid resuscitation are the main goals of managing rhabdomyolysis. When rhabdomyolysis is treated promptly and appropriately, the prognosis is usually good, especially in children.

The underlying reason and the efficacy of treatments for the underlying cause may have an impact on the prognosis and long-term consequences in cases with recurrent bouts of rhabdomyolysis, which may be indicative of problems in muscle structure or metabolism. Identifying and treating the underlying risk factors, such as limiting excessive physical activity, maintaining hydration, tracking and controlling medication, treating underlying infections and metabolic problems, and abstaining from alcohol and illegal drugs, are examples of preventive strategies. The common causes, diagnosis, and available treatments for rhabdomyolysis should be understood by all practitioners.

Reference

Rhabdomyolysis: Pathogenesis, Diagnosis, and Treatment - ResearchGate. (https://www.researchgate.net/publication/274401632_Rhabdomyolysis_Pathogenesis_Diagnosis_and_Treatment)

Rhabdomyolysis: An evidence-based approach - Sarah Burgess, 2022 - Sage Journals. (http://journals.sagepub.com/doi/10.1177/17514437211050782)

Rhabdomyolysis: pathogenesis, diagnosis, and treatment - PubMed. (https://pubmed.ncbi.nlm.nih.gov/25829882/)

Rhabdomyolysis: pathogenesis, diagnosis, and treatment - Semantic Scholar.

(https://www.semanticscholar.org/paper/Rhab
domyolysis%3A-pathogenesis%2C-diagnosis%2
C-and-Torres-Helmstetter/0f328bb0dfd1922b1
191303e055978422df45763)

About The Author

Murphy Green is an experienced medical practitioner and author who has dedicated years to the study and treatment of rhabdomyolysis. Their work encompasses an evidence-based approach to the diagnosis and management of rhabdomyolysis, as well as a comprehensive understanding of the condition's pathogenesis, diagnosis, and treatment. Green's expertise is evident in their contributions to the literature, including a review that focuses on the epidemiology, pathophysiology, causes, presentation, diagnosis, complications, management, and anesthetic considerations related to rhabdomyolysis. This extensive involvement in the field of rhabdomyolysis underscores Green's commitment to advancing the understanding and treatment of this condition, ultimately contributing to improved patient outcomes and the dissemination of valuable knowledge within the medical community.

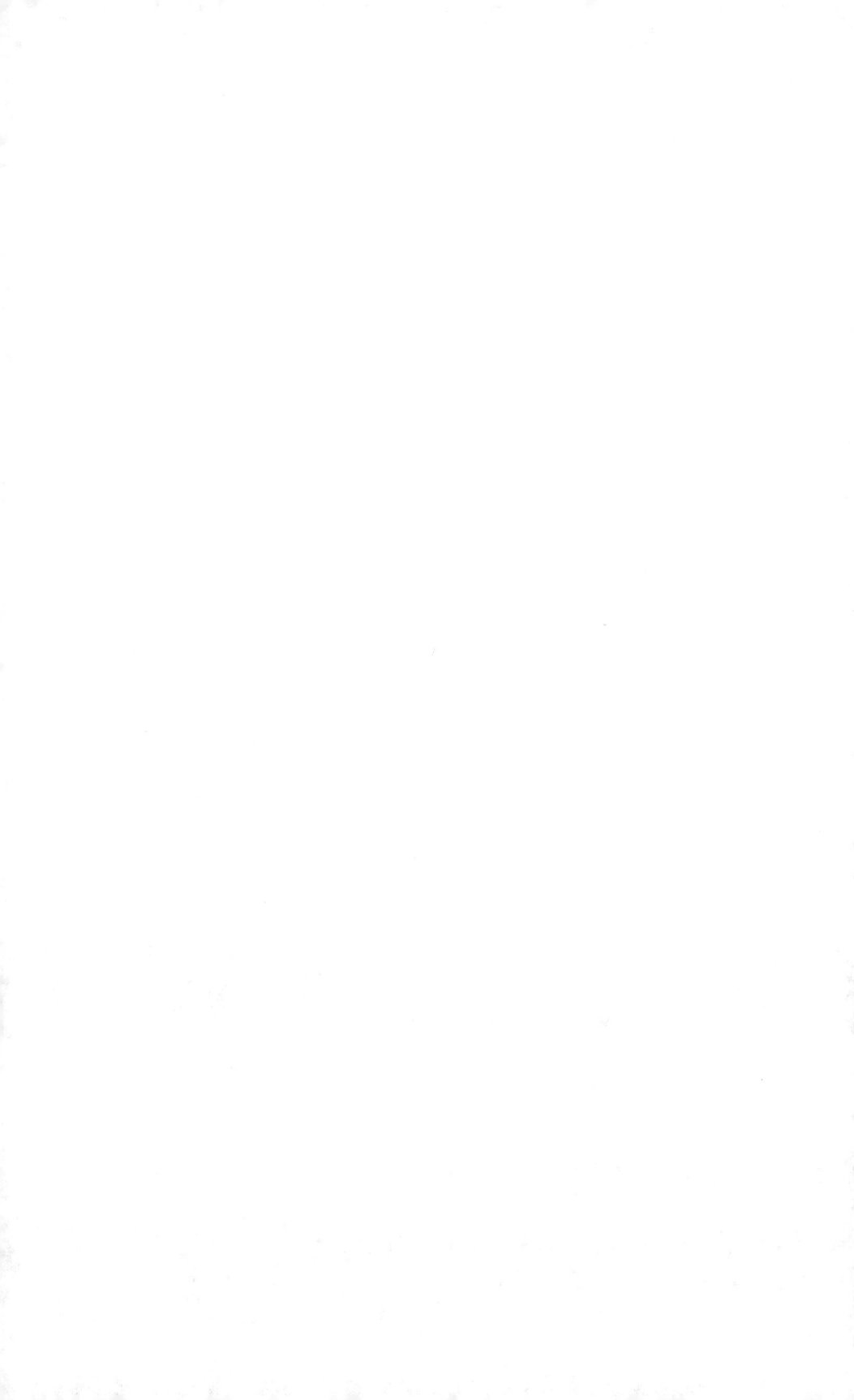